Breast Cancer Diaries

Inspirational Quotes, Thoughts and Comments

By

Dr. Charley Ferrer

Publisher
Cancer Tamer, Inc.
PO Box 140996
Staten Island NY 10314
info@cancerTamer.org
718-916-4124

ISBN 978-0-9982202-6-0 (Digital ISBN)
ISBN 978-0-9982202-5-3 (Paperback ISBN)

Book layout: Concierge Self-Publishing

This book is full of inspirational quotes by various individuals throughout history and present time. No claim is made to their copyright of the phrases or quotes, except for those attributed to Dr. Charley Ferrer whose inspirational quotes, thoughts, and comments are meant to encourage and challenge you to reach out and grasp your full potential splendor.

www.CancerTamer.org

You've heard those three little words which changed your life forever, "you have cancer."

Well, here are a few more words which I hope will change your life once more.

This time, bringing you a little joy, laughter, and a bit of inspiration to keep you going during this interesting journey we're on.

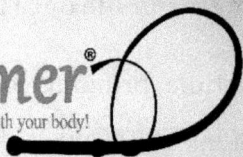

Cancer Tamer®
because you shouldn't be at war with your body!

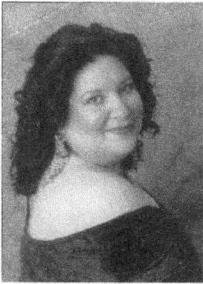

A Special Note
from
Dr. Charley Ferrer

When I was first diagnosed with breast cancer, I didn't expect the insanity it would bring into my life nor the new direction my life would take. I went from teaching others how to feel comfortable with themselves and their bodies, to experiencing a major body issue after my breast cancer surgeries.

In the months following my diagnosis, I became an avid reader on all things related to breast cancer and was obsessed with obtaining as much information as possible in the hopes it would alleviate my fears and help me gain a modicum of control in my life once more.

After the initial fear dissipated, I searched for books which would help keep me grounded and inspire me so the challenges I faced would not devastate me. I found some fabulous inspirational books and added them to the vast pile of others I had enjoyed in years gone by. (Several of these books are available on my website.)

I will admit, I love reading authors who challenge me to think, to grow, and to give myself a good swift kick in the ass when I'm wallowing in negativity and depression and not reaching out for my full potential. I would meticulously write down the marvelous secrets each book held, making connections and interpretations of my own. I would ponder the thoughts I resonated with and even more so those that challenged me; those that pushed me to step out of my comfort zone and demand more out of life.

Throughout these pages, I will share some of those *Inspirational Quotes, Thoughts and Comments*, a few connections I made, and challenge you with a few comments to consider for yourself. It is my hope these pages will inspire you and make you smile as you walk along the path of breast cancer which at times can be arduous; yet, also holds the potential for your greatest victories.

I've purposely structured *Breast Cancer Diaries: Inspirational Quotes, Thoughts and Comments* to be used as a journal—an inspirational workbook, if you will—for you to jot down the thoughts each quote, thought or comment awakens in you. It is my hope that doing so will lead you to many triumphs and lend you strength and laughter in the days ahead.

This book contains quotes and sayings, which I believe will help open your mind to new possibilities and higher levels of intuition and awakening. Choose a new quote each day and discover the meaning it holds for you. Look at it from all angles. Jot down your thoughts. Meditate on them. Record your thoughts on your smart phone to consider in more depth later. Allow yourself to make connections, assumptions, and consider new possibilities. Place no limitations—

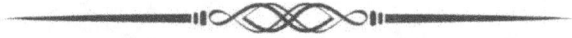

or judgements—on your thoughts or the connections you make. Allow your heart and mind to roam free. I truly believe that in doing this, you will find a measure of peace, hope, and even a sense of wonder, as you reach for your life's fullest potential. (The printed version of this book is an actual journal book with lined pages for you to write in.)

I've included 365 Inspirational Quotes, Thoughts and Comments in this book to carry you through a year's worth of growth and health. It doesn't matter when you start this book, or whether you go in order or jump around to passages you enjoy more, it only matters that you start and continue.

Use *Breast Cancer Diaries: Inspirational Quotes, Thoughts and Comments* to get you started in the morning, motivate you in the afternoon, or give you something to ponder before going to bed. Remember there is inspiration all around you, you merely need to open your heart and mind to it because life isn't merely surviving, it's about thriving!

Please feel free to share your thoughts and comments with me on our Facebook Group Page, Cancer Tamer, or through our website or email. I'd love to hear how *Breast Cancer Diaries: Inspirational Quotes, Thoughts and Comments* has impacted your life.

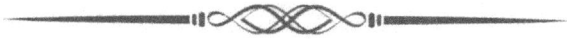

Live with ROARING passion,
Dr. Charley Ferrer

PS: If you wish to continue to be challenged and expand your mind further, perhaps even see life through a different lens, as you continue your path toward your full potential, check out the second book in this series, *Breast Cancer Diaries: Choose.*

All that we are is what we thought.

Buddha

_____

_____

_____

_____

_____

_____

_____

_____

_____

_____

_____

_____

_____

_____

_____

_____

_____

———— ⅠⅠ∞◇◇◇∞ⅠⅠ ————

You are a Badass!

Jen Sincero

_____

_____

_____

_____

_____

_____

_____

_____

_____

_____

_____

_____

_____

_____

_____

_____

_____

_____

Shine like the whole world is yours.

Rumi

_____

_____

_____

_____

_____

_____

_____

_____

_____

_____

_____

_____

_____

_____

_____

_____

Thoughts become things ...
choose the good ones!

Mike Dooley

Hope is being able to see that there is light
despite all of the darkness.

Desmond Tutu

———————⊪∝⟨✕⟩∽⊪———————

What if the world's greatest lie
was that at a certain point in our lives,
we lose control of what we want
and are then controlled by fate?

The Alchemist
Paulo Coelho

_____

_____

_____

_____

_____

_____

_____

_____

_____

_____

_____

_____

_____

_____

We do not need magic to change the world,
we carry the power we need inside
ourselves already: we have the power
to imagine better.

J.K. Rowling

———————||◦◇◇◇◦||———————

Follow your bliss and the universe
will open doors where once
there was only walls.

Joseph Campbell

_____

_____

_____

_____

_____

_____

_____

_____

_____

_____

_____

_____

_____

_____

_____

_____

_____

Where the willingness is great
the difficulties cannot be great.

Niccolo Machiavelli

_____

_____

_____

_____

_____

_____

_____

_____

_____

_____

_____

_____

_____

_____

_____

_____

_____

Negativity clouds your judgment
and stops you from living up
to your full potential.

Dr. Charley Ferrer

_____

_____

_____

_____

_____

_____

_____

_____

_____

_____

_____

_____

_____

_____

_____

We should expect the impossible.

James Baldwin

_____

_____

_____

_____

_____

_____

_____

_____

_____

_____

_____

_____

_____

_____

_____

_____

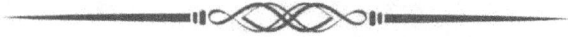

Do. The. Work.

Every day, you have to do something you don't want to do. Every day. Challenge yourself to be uncomfortable, push past the apathy and laziness and fear. Otherwise, the next day you're going to have two things you don't want to do, then three and four and five, and pretty soon, you can't even get back to the first thing. And then all you can do is beat yourself up for the mess you've created, and now you've got a mental barrier to go along with the physical barriers.

Relentless: From Good to Great
To Unstoppable
Tim S. Grover

_____

_____

_____

_____

It's not the light at the end of the tunnel
that's an illusion ... it's the tunnel.

Hemal Radia

_____

_____

_____

_____

_____

_____

_____

_____

_____

_____

_____

_____

_____

_____

_____

We're afraid of pain—we all are. But, all the good stuff—all the wisdom and courage we need to become the people we need to be next—is actually inside the pain.

Glennon Moyle Delton

———————110⋈∞⋈011———————

STOP surviving and START thriving!

Dr. Charley Ferrer

_____

_____

_____

_____

_____

_____

_____

_____

_____

_____

_____

_____

_____

_____

_____

If you think taking care of yourself
is selfish, change your mind.
If you don't, you're simply ducking
your responsibilities.

Ann Richards

_____

_____

_____

_____

_____

_____

_____

_____

_____

_____

_____

_____

_____

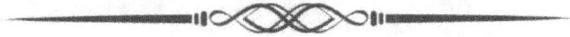

Today, at church, we were asked to stand up if we are grateful for something: some said they were grateful to be able to wake up today. Others were grateful to be able to breathe, eat, and laugh. I said, I was grateful that God has been watching over me, healing me, and keeping my family with me. Keep on praying.

Debra Santulli-Barone

If you only focus on the problem, you might
miss the solution.

Common Adage

_____

_____

_____

_____

_____

_____

_____

_____

_____

_____

_____

_____

_____

_____

_____

_____

_____

I choose to make the rest of my life
the best of my life.

Louise Hay

_____

_____

_____

_____

_____

_____

_____

_____

_____

_____

_____

_____

_____

_____

A great deal of talent is lost to the world for
want of a little courage.

Sidney Smith

_____

_____

_____

_____

_____

_____

_____

_____

_____

_____

_____

_____

_____

_____

_____

_____

_____

Use failure as a steppingstone to your
success not as an excuse to give up.

Maxwell Stone

It may be that when we no longer know
what to do, we have come to our real work
and when we no longer know which way to
go, we have begun our real journey.

Wendell Berry

Sin is anything one does or thinks that
causes them to be unhappy.

Outwitting the Devil
Napoleon Hill

_____

_____

_____

_____

_____

_____

_____

_____

_____

_____

_____

_____

_____

_____

_____

_____

Change your thoughts
and you change your world.

Norman Vincent Peale

_____

_____

_____

_____

_____

_____

_____

_____

_____

_____

_____

_____

_____

_____

_____

_____

_____

In order to be irreplaceable,
one must always be different.

Coco Chanel

Don't compromise yourself.
You are all you've got.
There is no yesterday, no tomorrow,
it's all the same day.

Janis Joplin, Singer

_____

_____

_____

_____

_____

_____

_____

_____

_____

_____

_____

_____

_____

_____

Find something ... just one small something ...
every day that makes your heart
sing for just a second.

Dr. Charley Ferrer

_____

_____

_____

_____

_____

_____

_____

_____

_____

_____

_____

_____

_____

_____

_____

Find your joy and live it.

The Secret
Rhonda Byrne

_____

_____

_____

_____

_____

_____

_____

_____

_____

_____

_____

_____

_____

_____

_____

_____

Say only what you want to be true because
life might be listening.

The Alchemist
Paulo Coelho

_____

_____

_____

_____

_____

_____

_____

_____

_____

_____

_____

_____

_____

_____

_____

You cannot always choose how you feel
but you can control how you act.

Mel Robbins

_____
_____
_____
_____
_____
_____
_____
_____
_____
_____
_____
_____
_____
_____
_____
_____

Worry is a form of praying
for what you don't want.

Common Axiom

_____

_____

_____

_____

_____

_____

_____

_____

_____

_____

_____

_____

_____

_____

_____

_____

_____

Claim your greatness.

Gary John Bishop

_____

_____

_____

_____

_____

_____

_____

_____

_____

_____

_____

_____

_____

_____

_____

_____

_____

_____

———||◇◇◇||———

There is no will power --
there's only choice.
What is yours?

Dr. Charley Ferrer

_____
_____
_____
_____
_____
_____
_____
_____
_____
_____
_____
_____
_____
_____
_____

Things of value require sacrifice. If people are too hurt, too busy or too damn stupid to see that you're a blessing they've been asking for, just fall back. Know your worth.

Anonymous

_____

_____

_____

_____

_____

_____

_____

_____

_____

_____

_____

_____

_____

_____

_____

Don't cry because it's over,
smile because it happened.

Dr. Seuss

Clouds don't worry about
falling into the sea because
they can't (a) fall or (b) drown.
But they are free
to believe they can,
and they may fear
if they wish.

Messiah's Handbook
Reminders for the Advanced Soul
Richard Bach

_____

_____

_____

_____

_____

_____

_____

_____

_____

_____

Don't forget you're human.

It's okay to have a meltdown.

Just don't unpack and live there. Cry it out.

Then refocus on where you're headed

Unknown

Two things are infinite:
the universe and human stupidity;
and I'm not sure about the universe.

Albert Einstein

_____
_____
_____
_____
_____
_____
_____
_____
_____
_____
_____
_____
_____
_____
_____
_____
_____

When opportunity presents itself, grab it.
Hold on tight and don't let go.

Celia Cruz, Singer

_____

_____

_____

_____

_____

_____

_____

_____

_____

_____

_____

_____

_____

_____

_____

_____

—————————||∽◇◇◇◇∽||—————————

The only thing worse than being blind
is having sight but no vision.

Helen Keller

_____

_____

_____

_____

_____

_____

_____

_____

_____

_____

_____

_____

_____

_____

_____

_____

_____

_____

Many men have robbed themselves of their
destiny because they allowed
discouragement to rob them
of their dreams.

The Legend of the Monk and The Merchant
Terry Felber

_____

_____

_____

_____

_____

_____

_____

_____

_____

_____

_____

_____

_____

_____

Strong women don't play the victim.
Don't make themselves look pitiful
and don't point fingers.
They stand and they deal.

Mandy Hale

_____

_____

_____

_____

_____

_____

_____

_____

_____

_____

_____

_____

_____

_____

Everybody dies ... but not everybody lives.

_____

_____

_____

_____

_____

_____

_____

_____

_____

_____

_____

_____

_____

_____

_____

_____

_____

Why do we need to wait for Christmas, holidays, birthdays or special occasions to give presents? Love and affection should be shared any time.

Dr. Charley Ferrer

Do not destroy your future
merely to get through today.

Unknown

Cancer is simply the symptom
and NOT the cause.

_____

_____

_____

_____

_____

_____

_____

_____

_____

_____

_____

_____

_____

_____

_____

_____

_____

———ıı∘⟨⟨⟩⟩∘ıı———

Live. Love. Dance.

Debra Santulli-Barone

_____
_____
_____
_____
_____
_____
_____
_____
_____
_____
_____
_____
_____
_____
_____
_____
_____

———||◁◆◆▷||———

Only the stupid regret choices.
The smart learn to adapt.

Nalini Singh, Author

_____

_____

_____

_____

_____

_____

_____

_____

_____

_____

_____

_____

_____

_____

_____

_____

_____

The mark of your ignorance is the depth of
your belief in injustice and tragedy.
What a caterpillar believed is the end of the
world, the master calls a butterfly.

Illusions
Richard Bach

_____

_____

_____

_____

_____

_____

_____

_____

_____

_____

_____

_____

_____

━━━━━━━⊪∞◇∞⊩━━━━━━━

Good enough NEVER is.

Debbie Fields

_____

_____

_____

_____

_____

_____

_____

_____

_____

_____

_____

_____

_____

_____

_____

_____

_____

Choose

Dr. Charley Ferrer

_____

_____

_____

_____

_____

_____

_____

_____

_____

_____

_____

_____

_____

_____

_____

_____

_____

_____

You must think you are more
than what you think you are.

Power of Decisions
Raymond Charles Barker

_____

_____

_____

_____

_____

_____

_____

_____

_____

_____

_____

_____

_____

_____

_____

_____

When one door of happiness closes, another opens; but often we look so long at the closed door that we do not see the one which has been opened for us.

Helen Keller

———————— ll∞◇◇◇∞ll ————————

Don't be a drifter on the sea of life.

Unknown

_____

_____

_____

_____

_____

_____

_____

_____

_____

_____

_____

_____

_____

_____

_____

_____

_____

Consider and act with reference to the true
ends of existence. This world is but the
vestibule of an immortal life. Every action
of our lives touches on some chord
that will vibrate in eternity.

Edwin Hubbell Chapin

_____
_____
_____
_____
_____
_____
_____
_____
_____
_____
_____
_____
_____

———————— ⅱ◦⟨⟩◦ⅱ ————————

Go from confused and frightened
to confident and in control by getting
educated and begin to reclaim control of
your life by taking responsibility
and an active role in your own
health and treatment.

Dr. Charley Ferrer

_____

_____

_____

_____

_____

_____

_____

_____

_____

_____

_____

_____

Once you reach the summit of your own
heart you will see beauty is everywhere.

Bryant McGill

There are a thousand thousand reasons to
live this life, every one of them sufficient.

Gilead
Marilynne Robinson

_____
_____
_____
_____
_____
_____
_____
_____
_____
_____
_____
_____
_____
_____
_____
_____

When the whole world is silent,
even one voice becomes powerful.

Malala Yousafzai

Imperfection is beauty,
madness is genius
and it's better to be absolutely ridiculous
than absolutely boring.

Marilyn Monroe

What they say or think
doesn't change your masterpiece.

Joel Osteen

Holding onto resentment is like taking
poison and waiting for your enemy to die.

Nelson Mandela

_____

_____

_____

_____

_____

_____

_____

_____

_____

_____

_____

_____

_____

_____

_____

_____

_____

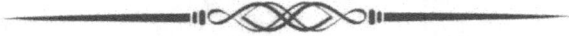

Our deepest fear is that we are
powerful beyond measure.
It is our light, not our darkness
that most frightens us.
Your playing small does not serve the world.
There is nothing enlightened about shrinking
so that other people won't feel
insecure around you.

Marianne Williamson

_____

_____

_____

_____

_____

_____

_____

_____

_____

_____

Money is like water flowing
down the river. Will you have a puddle
or a river at the bottom?

Unknown

_____

_____

_____

_____

_____

_____

_____

_____

_____

_____

_____

_____

_____

_____

Power is like being a lady,
if you have to tell people you are,
you aren't.

Margaret Thatcher

In three words I can sum up everything
I've learned about life:
it goes on.

Robert Frost

_____

_____

_____

_____

_____

_____

_____

_____

_____

_____

_____

_____

_____

_____

_____

Don't walk in front of me ...
I may not follow.
Don't walk behind me ... I may not lead.
Walk beside me ... just be my friend.

Albert Camus

_____

_____

_____

_____

_____

_____

_____

_____

_____

_____

_____

_____

_____

You create your own destiny with your
thoughts. Get clear about what you want.
Know what you want.
Believe
—you must believe—
what you asked for you will receive.

Dr. Charley Ferrer

_____
_____
_____
_____
_____
_____
_____
_____
_____
_____
_____
_____
_____

Don't be afraid to go where you've
never gone and do what you've never done,
because both are necessary
to have what you've never had
and be who you've never been.

Notes from the Universe
Mike Dooley

_____

_____

_____

_____

_____

_____

_____

_____

_____

_____

_____

_____

_____

_____

Better than the deed.
Better than the memory.
It's the moment of anticipation.

The Simpsons
Matt Groening

_____

_____

_____

_____

_____

_____

_____

_____

_____

_____

_____

_____

_____

———=||◇◇◇◇◇||=———

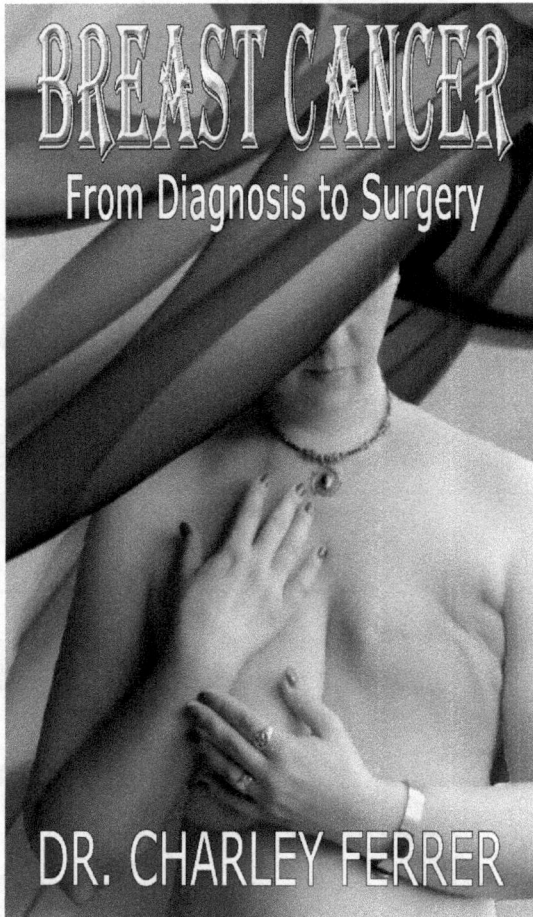

BREAST CANCER
From Diagnosis to Surgery

DR. CHARLEY FERRER

Don't settle for what you can get,
INSTEAD
create what you want!

Dr. Charley Ferrer

_____

_____

_____

_____

_____

_____

_____

_____

_____

_____

_____

_____

_____

_____

_____

_____

Before the truth can set you free
you need to recognize which lie
is holding you hostage.

Rachel Wolchin

To hell with circumstances
I create circumstance.

Patricia G. Horn

_____

_____

_____

_____

_____

_____

_____

_____

_____

_____

_____

_____

_____

_____

_____

_____

_____

The two most important days in your life
are the day you were born
and the day you find out why.

Mark Twain

_____

_____

_____

_____

_____

_____

_____

_____

_____

_____

_____

_____

_____

_____

_____

Money is about what you believe you
deserve and can have for yourself.

Dr. Charley Ferrer

_____

_____

_____

_____

_____

_____

_____

_____

_____

_____

_____

_____

_____

_____

_____

_____

_____

No man is good enough to govern
any woman without her consent.

Susan B. Anthony

———————————— Ⅱ◇◇◇◇ Ⅱ ————————————

Those who cannot [and do not]
remember the past are condemned to repeat it.

George Santayana
1863 – 1952

_____

_____

_____

_____

_____

_____

_____

_____

_____

_____

_____

_____

_____

_____

_____

My first American experience was in the harbor of New York City when I saw that amazing big, tall lady. I remember thinking, "Oh my goodness, a lady runs this country."

Rita Moreno

Baby souls follow. Young souls lead. But old souls are just as happy to dance alone.

Notes from the Universe
Mike Dooley

_____

_____

_____

_____

_____

_____

_____

_____

_____

_____

_____

_____

_____

_____

_____

_____

===||◇◇◇||===

If you ever get bored, just open your eyes.

Liven Rosset

_____

_____

_____

_____

_____

_____

_____

_____

_____

_____

_____

_____

_____

_____

_____

_____

_____

_____

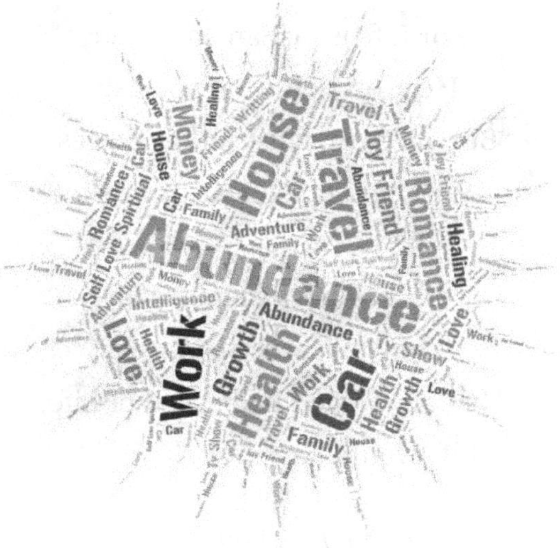
Abundance
Work
Car
Health
House
Travel
Romance
Money
Joy Friend
Love
Healing
Growth
Family
Adventure
Intelligence
Self Love Spiritual
Tv Show

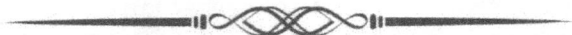

I bargained with Life for a penny,
And Life would pay no more,
However I begged at evening
When I counted my scanty store;

For Life is just an employer,
He gives you what you ask,
But once you have set the wages,
Why, you must bear the task.

I worked for a menial's hire,
Only to learn, dismayed,
That any wage I had asked of Life,
Life would have [surely] paid.

Jessie B. Rittenhouse

_____

_____

_____

_____

We travel not to escape life,
but for life not to escape us.

Anonymous

_____

_____

_____

_____

_____

_____

_____

_____

_____

_____

_____

_____

_____

_____

_____

_____

You have been assigned this mountain so
you can show others it can be moved.

Mel Robbins

_____

_____

_____

_____

_____

_____

_____

_____

_____

_____

_____

_____

_____

_____

_____

_____

_____

In a car, the windshield is big so you can see where you're going. The rear view mirror is small, because where you've been isn't as important as where you're going.

Joel Osteen

_____

_____

_____

_____

_____

_____

_____

_____

_____

_____

_____

_____

_____

_____

What is deemed as "his-story"
is often determined by those
who survived to write it.

Boudicca
Celtic Queen & Warrior
(circa 30 – 61 AD)

_____

_____

_____

_____

_____

_____

_____

_____

_____

_____

_____

_____

_____

_____

There is power in responsibility.

Tony Robbins

_____

_____

_____

_____

_____

_____

_____

_____

_____

_____

_____

_____

_____

_____

_____

_____

Excited misery.

Melody Beattie

_____
_____
_____
_____
_____
_____
_____
_____
_____
_____
_____
_____
_____
_____
_____
_____

There's a major difference between
"have to" and "choose to."
Which are you focused on?

Dr. Charley Ferrer

_____

_____

_____

_____

_____

_____

_____

_____

_____

_____

_____

_____

_____

_____

Let go of what's holding you back
so you can reach for what you want.

Miranda Bailey—Grey's Anatomy
Shonda Rhimes

Judgments are like mud;
you can get covered by them
or you can walk around the dirt
to get to the other side.

Dr. Charley Ferrer

_____

_____

_____

_____

_____

_____

_____

_____

_____

_____

_____

_____

_____

_____

_____

_____

If you want your life to be different,
you have to make it happen.

Gary John Bishop

_____

_____

_____

_____

_____

_____

_____

_____

_____

_____

_____

_____

_____

_____

There are no limitations to the mind except
those you acknowledge.

Napoleon Hill

_____

_____

_____

_____

_____

_____

_____

_____

_____

_____

_____

_____

_____

_____

_____

_____

_____

———·II◦◇◇◦II·———

Write it on your heart
that every day
is the best day of the year.

Ralph Waldo Emerson

_____

_____

_____

_____

_____

_____

_____

_____

_____

_____

_____

_____

_____

_____

Walking in the dark with a friend
is better than walking in the light alone.

Helen Keller

_____

_____

_____

_____

_____

_____

_____

_____

_____

_____

_____

_____

_____

_____

_____

_____

_____

_____

All our dreams can come true,
if we have the courage to pursue them.

Walt Disney

You can waste your life drawing lines.
Or you can live your life crossing them.

Shonda Rhimes

_____

_____

_____

_____

_____

_____

_____

_____

_____

_____

_____

_____

_____

_____

_____

The way we talk to our children
becomes their inner voice.

Peggy O'Mara

Yesterday is not ours to recover,
but tomorrow is ours to win or lose.

Lyndon B. Johnson

_____

_____

_____

_____

_____

_____

_____

_____

_____

_____

_____

_____

_____

_____

_____

_____

_____

_____

Don't think about where you are today,
think about where you're going
to be tomorrow.

Taffy Blacker
South Africa

_____

_____

_____

_____

_____

_____

_____

_____

_____

_____

_____

_____

_____

You know you're in love
when you can't fall asleep
because reality is finally better
than your dreams.

Dr. Seuss

_____

_____

_____

_____

_____

_____

_____

_____

_____

_____

_____

_____

_____

_____

_____

To find yourself, think for yourself.

Socrates

Honesty and transparency
make you vulnerable.
Be honest and transparent anyway.

Mother Theresa

_____

_____

_____

_____

_____

_____

_____

_____

_____

_____

_____

_____

_____

_____

_____

_____

No one man can, for any considerable time,
wear one face to himself, and another to the
multitude, without finally getting bewildered
as to which is the true one.

Nathaniel Hawthorne

_____

_____

_____

_____

_____

_____

_____

_____

_____

_____

_____

_____

_____

_____

_____

The difference between successful people
and others is how long they spend time
feeling sorry for themselves.

Barbara Corcoran

_____

_____

_____

_____

_____

_____

_____

_____

_____

_____

_____

_____

_____

_____

_____

The privilege of a lifetime
is to become who you truly are.

Carl Jung

Forget conventionalisms; forget what the
world thinks of you stepping out of your
place; think your best thoughts, speak your
best words, work your best works, looking
to your own conscience for approval.

Susan B. Anthony

_____

_____

_____

_____

_____

_____

_____

_____

_____

_____

_____

_____

_____

Everything will line up perfectly when
knowing and living the truth becomes more
important than looking good.

Alan Cohen

_____
_____
_____
_____
_____
_____
_____
_____
_____
_____
_____
_____
_____
_____
_____
_____

—————— ᛁᛁ◇◇◇ᛁᛁ ——————

Never make a major decision in a valley.

Three Feet from Gold
Sharon L. Lechter & Greg S. Reid

_____

_____

_____

_____

_____

_____

_____

_____

_____

_____

_____

_____

_____

_____

_____

_____

_____

You only live once,
but if you do it right,
once is enough.

Mae West

Love the one you IS.

Hay House

_____

_____

_____

_____

_____

_____

_____

_____

_____

_____

_____

_____

_____

_____

_____

_____

_____

_____

_____

To make a difference in someone's life
you don't have to be brilliant,
rich, beautiful or perfect.
You just have to care.

Mandy Hale

The kite flies against the wind not with it.

Napoleon Hill

You have one true job in life ...
to love yourself for all you are
and all you are meant to be.

Financial prosperity is often
connected to soul prosperity.

The Legend of the Monk and The Merchant
Terry Felber

_____

_____

_____

_____

_____

_____

_____

_____

_____

_____

_____

_____

_____

_____

_____

_____

_____

Everybody's got a past. The past does not
equal the future unless you live there.

Tony Robbins

_____

_____

_____

_____

_____

_____

_____

_____

_____

_____

_____

_____

_____

_____

_____

_____

_____

_____

Everyone has inside of her a piece of good news.
The good news is that you don't know
how great you can be, how much you can
love, what you can accomplish, and what
your potential is.

Anne Frank

_____

_____

_____

_____

_____

_____

_____

_____

_____

_____

_____

_____

_____

An excuse is just a challenge
you've given your power to.

Jen Sincero

Don't nourish your fears more
than you nourish your hopes.

Steve Maraboli

_____

_____

_____

_____

_____

_____

_____

_____

_____

_____

_____

_____

_____

_____

_____

_____

_____

_____

If your goals aren't making you
lick your lips, they're not big enough!

Hemal Radia

I might be hurting
but I'm still in the game!

Dr. Charley Ferrer

_____

_____

_____

_____

_____

_____

_____

_____

_____

_____

_____

_____

_____

_____

_____

_____

_____

God meets you at the level of your prayers ...
so pray BIG!

_____

_____

_____

_____

_____

_____

_____

_____

_____

_____

_____

_____

_____

_____

_____

_____

_____

_____

_____

You can never leave footprints that last
if you are always walking on tiptoe.

Leymah Gbowee

_____

_____

_____

_____

_____

_____

_____

_____

_____

_____

_____

_____

_____

_____

_____

_____

_____

_____

Heaven is about abundance.

It's about manifesting your desires.

It's you're right!

You can't ever get enough.

Believe it ... it's true.

You can't bankrupt Heaven!

So ask for all you desire.

Manifest all your dreams.

Live life.

It was created for you.

Dr. Charley Ferrer

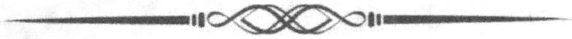

_____

_____

_____

_____

_____

_____

_____

_____

———————

Meaning isn't something you find,
it's something you give.

The Closer
Television Series

_____

_____

_____

_____

_____

_____

_____

_____

_____

_____

_____

_____

_____

_____

_____

Perception creates reality.

Barbara Corcoran

Excuses don't build Empires.

Daymond John

_____

_____

_____

_____

_____

_____

_____

_____

_____

_____

_____

_____

_____

_____

_____

_____

_____

_____

———II○◇◇◇○II———

Fear is NOT the only option!

Dr. Charley Ferrer

_____

_____

_____

_____

_____

_____

_____

_____

_____

_____

_____

_____

_____

_____

_____

_____

_____

_____

I am a woman with thoughts and questions
and shit to say. I say if I'm beautiful. I say
if I'm strong. You will not determine my
story—I will.

Amy Schumer

If you don't take care of this magnificent machine
you were given (your body),
where are you going to live?

Karyn Calabrese

Change your imagination
and you change the world

Neville Goddard

_____

_____

_____

_____

_____

_____

_____

_____

_____

_____

_____

_____

_____

_____

_____

_____

_____

_____

Presence is more important than
performance. People don't always remember
what you said, but they remember
how you made them feel.

Maya Angelou

_____

_____

_____

_____

_____

_____

_____

_____

_____

_____

_____

_____

_____

———— ‖◇◇◇‖ ————

A bird doesn't sing because it has an
answer, it sings because it has a song.

Joan Walsh Anglund

_____

_____

_____

_____

_____

_____

_____

_____

_____

_____

_____

_____

_____

_____

_____

_____

Beliefs and thoughts
alter the cells in your body.

Bruce Lipton
Father of Epigenetics

_____

_____

_____

_____

_____

_____

_____

_____

_____

_____

_____

_____

_____

_____

Wake up and kick ass!

Kicking Horse Coffee

_____

_____

_____

_____

_____

_____

_____

_____

_____

_____

_____

_____

_____

_____

_____

_____

Your body hears everything
your mind says.

Naomi Judd

Money isn't everything
but it ranks right up there with oxygen.

Rita Davenport

_____

_____

_____

_____

_____

_____

_____

_____

_____

_____

_____

_____

_____

_____

_____

_____

Favor is the fog

through which we collapse triumph.

Aldrich Killian
Iron Man III

_____

_____

_____

_____

_____

_____

_____

_____

_____

_____

_____

_____

_____

_____

I declare to you that woman must not
depend upon the protection of man,
but must be taught to protect herself,
and there I take my stand.

Susan B. Anthony

We create our own demons.
Therefore, we know the secrets
to destroying them.

Dr. Charley Ferrer

_____

_____

_____

_____

_____

_____

_____

_____

_____

_____

_____

_____

_____

_____

If you don't like the road you're walking,
start paving another one.

Dolly Parton, Singer

_____

_____

_____

_____

_____

_____

_____

_____

_____

_____

_____

_____

_____

_____

_____

My mission in life is not merely to survive,
but to thrive; and to do so with some
passion, some compassion, some humor,
and some style.

Maya Angelou

_____

_____

_____

_____

_____

_____

_____

_____

_____

_____

_____

_____

_____

_____

Life shrinks or expands
in proportion to one's courage.

Anais Nin

_____

_____

_____

_____

_____

_____

_____

_____

_____

_____

_____

_____

_____

_____

_____

_____

Life begins
at the end of your comfort zone.

Neale Donald Walsch

Broke is temporary. Poor is eternal.

Rich Dad Poor Dad
Sharon L. Lechter & Robert T. Klyosaki

_____

_____

_____

_____

_____

_____

_____

_____

_____

_____

_____

_____

_____

_____

_____

_____

Yesterday's pains

is the Warrior of the Light's strength.

The Warrior of the Light
Paulo Coelho

_____

_____

_____

_____

_____

_____

_____

_____

_____

_____

_____

_____

_____

_____

Impossible
is self-imposed limitations
you create in yourself.

Unexpected
are possibilities
you hadn't yet thought of.

_____

_____

_____

_____

_____

_____

_____

_____

_____

_____

_____

_____

Sometimes when you're in a dark place,
you think you've been buried
but you've actually been planted.

Christine Caine

———————— ⅡⅭ◇◇◇Ⅱ ————————

Like the baby chick and the egg shell,
the real you is within.

Dr. Charley Ferrer

_____

_____

_____

_____

_____

_____

_____

_____

_____

_____

_____

_____

_____

_____

_____

_____

_____

One of the secrets to staying young is to always do things you don't know how to do, to keep learning.

Ruth Reichl

_____

_____

_____

_____

_____

_____

_____

_____

_____

_____

_____

_____

_____

_____

Face the lies of illness
with the truths of health.

The Power of Decision
Raymond Charles Barker

_____

_____

_____

_____

_____

_____

_____

_____

_____

_____

_____

_____

_____

_____

_____

_____

———— ❘❘◇◇◇◇◇◇◇◇❘❘ ————

You are a woman and you should decorate
yourself however it pleases you.

Julia to Plum on Dietland
Sarai Walker

_____

_____

_____

_____

_____

_____

_____

_____

_____

_____

_____

_____

_____

_____

I can't change the direction of the wind,
but I can adjust my sails
to always reach my destination.

Jimmy Dean

_____

_____

_____

_____

_____

_____

_____

_____

_____

_____

_____

_____

_____

_____

Look your best—who said love is blind?

Mae West

You don't have to be perfect
to make a difference.

_____

_____

_____

_____

_____

_____

_____

_____

_____

_____

_____

_____

_____

_____

_____

_____

Doubt creates doubt, lowers self-esteem, makes you question your self-worth, your actions and your abilities. Doubt will rationalize itself to help prove the negativity that surrounds it. Doubt can't exist in truth. Find your truth!

Dr. Charley Ferrer

_____

_____

_____

_____

_____

_____

_____

_____

_____

_____

_____

_____

It's not about being worthy.
It's about recognizing your worth.

Dr. Isaura Gonzalez

_____

_____

_____

_____

_____

_____

_____

_____

_____

_____

_____

_____

_____

_____

_____

_____

_____

Dr. Charley Ferrer

It took me quite a long time to develop
a voice, and now that I have it,
I am not going to be silent.

Madeleine Albright

_____
_____
_____
_____
_____
_____
_____
_____
_____
_____
_____
_____
_____
_____

I am the Master of my thoughts!
Rinse and repeat.

_____

_____

_____

_____

_____

_____

_____

_____

_____

_____

_____

_____

_____

_____

_____

_____

_____

_____

Love yourself. If not now, when?

Dr. Charley Ferrer

_____

_____

_____

_____

_____

_____

_____

_____

_____

_____

_____

_____

_____

_____

_____

_____

_____

We have nothing to fear but fear itself.

Franklin Delano Roosevelt

_____

_____

_____

_____

_____

_____

_____

_____

_____

_____

_____

_____

_____

_____

_____

_____

_____

_____

The more we know; the more we can do.

Dr. Andrew Well

_____

_____

_____

_____

_____

_____

_____

_____

_____

_____

_____

_____

_____

_____

_____

_____

———————◆———————

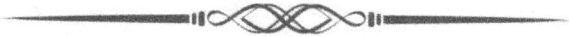

When I run after what I think I want,
my days are a furnace of stress and anxiety;
if I sit in my own place of patience,
what I need flows to me,
and without pain.

From this I understand that what I want
also wants me,
is looking for me
and attracting me.

There is a great secret here
for anyone who can grasp it.

Rumi

_____

_____

_____

_____

_____

========⊪◯⧄⧄◯⊪========

No one can make you feel inferior
without your consent.

Eleanor Roosevelt

_____

_____

_____

_____

_____

_____

_____

_____

_____

_____

_____

_____

_____

_____

_____

_____

_____

Breast Cancer Diaries: Inspirational Quotes,
Thoughts and Comments

If you tell the truth,
you don't have to remember anything.

Mark Twain

To live is the rarest thing in the world.
Most people exist, that is all.

Oscar Wilde

_____
_____
_____
_____
_____
_____
_____
_____
_____
_____
_____
_____
_____
_____
_____
_____
_____

What you do makes a difference,
and you have to decide what kind of
difference you want to make.

Jane Goodall

_____

_____

_____

_____

_____

_____

_____

_____

_____

_____

_____

_____

_____

_____

_____

_____

To be yourself in a world that is constantly
trying to make you something else
is the greatest accomplishment.

Ralph Waldo Emerson

We accept the love we think we deserve.

Stephen Chbosky

_____

_____

_____

_____

_____

_____

_____

_____

_____

_____

_____

_____

_____

_____

_____

_____

_____

_____

A reader lives a thousand lives before he dies, said Jojen. The man who never reads lives only one.

A Dance with Dragons
George R.R. Martin

_____

_____

_____

_____

_____

_____

_____

_____

_____

_____

_____

_____

The question isn't who is going to let me;
it's who is going to stop me.

Ayn Rand

_____

_____

_____

_____

_____

_____

_____

_____

_____

_____

_____

_____

_____

_____

_____

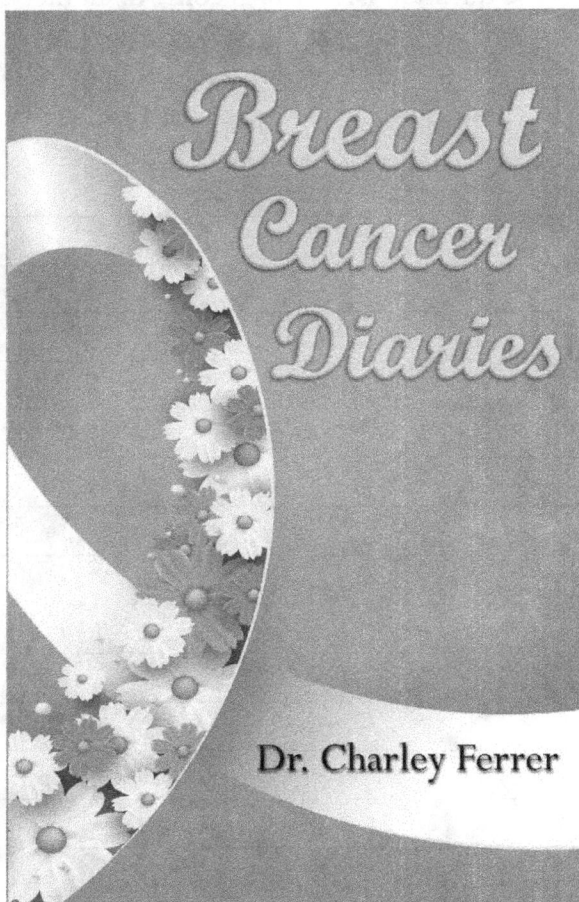

Breast Cancer Diaries

Dr. Charley Ferrer

Being deeply loved by someone gives you
strength, while loving someone deeply
gives you courage.

Lao Tzu

It is never too late to be what
you might have been.

George Eliot

_____
_____
_____
_____
_____
_____
_____
_____
_____
_____
_____
_____
_____
_____
_____
_____

Love is that condition in which the
happiness of another person
is essential to your own.

Stranger in a Strange Land
Robert A. Heinlein

_____

_____

_____

_____

_____

_____

_____

_____

_____

_____

_____

_____

_____

_____

Everything you can imagine is real.

Pablo Picasso

_____

_____

_____

_____

_____

_____

_____

_____

_____

_____

_____

_____

_____

_____

_____

_____

We don't see things as they are,
we see them as we are.

Anaïs Nin

_____

_____

_____

_____

_____

_____

_____

_____

_____

_____

_____

_____

_____

_____

_____

_____

The difference between genius and
stupidity is: genius has its limits.

Alexandre Dumas-fils

You are more powerful than you know;
you are beautiful just as you are.

Melissa Etheridge

_____

_____

_____

_____

_____

_____

_____

_____

_____

_____

_____

_____

_____

_____

_____

_____

_____

_____

A woman is the full circle. Within her is
the power to create, nurture and transform.

Diane Mariechild

_____

_____

_____

_____

_____

_____

_____

_____

_____

_____

_____

_____

_____

_____

_____

The most effective way to do it, is to do it.

Amelia Earhart

_____

_____

_____

_____

_____

_____

_____

_____

_____

_____

_____

_____

_____

_____

_____

_____

_____

_____

If you obey all the rules,
you miss all the fun.

Katharine Hepburn, Actress

Success is not final,
failure is not fatal:
it is the courage to continue that counts.

Winston S. Churchill

_____

_____

_____

_____

_____

_____

_____

_____

_____

_____

_____

_____

_____

_____

_____

Fear is a filter. A lie. An illusion.

Everything you want is behind the fear.

Fear is merely there to ensure

you really want "it."

If not, you'll walk away.

If you do want "it," you'll fight for "it"

and overcome your fear to obtain "it."

What is "it" for you?

Dr. Charley Ferrer

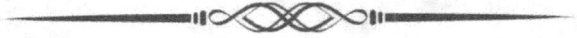

_____

_____

_____

_____

_____

_____

_____

_____

_____

_____

Our greatest glory is not in never falling,
but in rising every time we fall.

Confucius

_____

_____

_____

_____

_____

_____

_____

_____

_____

_____

_____

_____

_____

_____

_____

_____

Happiness is when what you think, what
you say, and what you do are in harmony.

Mahatma Gandhi

_____
_____
_____
_____
_____
_____
_____
_____
_____
_____
_____
_____
_____

No man is free who has not mastered himself.

Epictetus
(circa 55 – 135 AD)

And one day, she discovered that she was
fierce and strong, and full of fire and that not
even she could hold herself back because
her passion burned brighter than her fears.

Mark Anthony

———————◦◦◦◦◦———————

A person's health isn't generally a
reflection of genes, but how their
environment is influencing them.
Genes are the direct cause of less
than 1% of diseases; 99% is how
we respond to the world.

The Biology of Believe
Bruce Lipton

_____

_____

_____

_____

_____

_____

_____

_____

_____

_____

Everything you've ever wanted
is on the other side of fear.

George Addair

_____

_____

_____

_____

_____

_____

_____

_____

_____

_____

_____

_____

_____

_____

_____

_____

Hardships often prepare ordinary people
for an extraordinary destiny.

C.S. Lewis

_____

_____

_____

_____

_____

_____

_____

_____

_____

_____

_____

_____

_____

_____

_____

_____

_____

Believe in yourself. You are braver than
you think, more talented than you know, and
capable of more than you imagine.

Roy T. Bennett

Start by doing what's necessary;
then do what's possible;
and suddenly you are doing the impossible.

Francis of Assisi

_____

_____

_____

_____

_____

_____

_____

_____

_____

_____

_____

_____

_____

_____

_____

_____

I attribute my success to this:
I never gave or took any excuse.

Florence Nightingale

———◄◦◯◯◦►———

We can never see beyond
the choices we don't understand.

The Oracle
The Matrix Reloaded

_____

_____

_____

_____

_____

_____

_____

_____

_____

_____

_____

_____

_____

_____

_____

_____

_____

_____

Because one believes in oneself,
one doesn't try to convince others.
Because one is content with oneself,
one doesn't need others' approval.
Because one accepts oneself,
the whole world accepts him or her.

Lao Tzu

_____

_____

_____

_____

_____

_____

_____

_____

_____

_____

_____

As soon as you trust yourself,
you will know how to live.

Johann Wolfgang von Goethe

_____

_____

_____

_____

_____

_____

_____

_____

_____

_____

_____

_____

_____

_____

_____

_____

_____

With realization of one's own potential
and self-confidence in one's ability,
one can build a better world.

Dalai Lama

Life is too short to waste any amount of time on wondering what other people think about you. In the first place, if they had better things going on in their lives, they wouldn't have the time to sit around and talk about you. What's important to me is not others' opinions of me, but what's important to me is my opinion of myself.

C. Joybell C.

Life is not easy for any of us.
But what of that?
We must have perseverance and above all
confidence in ourselves. We must believe
that we are gifted for something,
and that this thing, at whatever cost,
must be attained.

Marie Curie

_____

_____

_____

_____

_____

_____

_____

_____

_____

_____

_____

If you want to improve your self-worth,
stop giving other people the calculator.

Tim Fargo

Dr. Charley Ferrer

We are what we believe we are.

C.S. Lewis

_____

_____

_____

_____

_____

_____

_____

_____

_____

_____

_____

_____

_____

_____

_____

_____

_____

_____

If you hear a voice within you say,
"you cannot paint,"
then by all means paint,
and that voice will be silenced.

Vincent van Gogh

_____

_____

_____

_____

_____

_____

_____

_____

_____

_____

_____

_____

_____

_____

Don't be satisfied with stories,
how things have gone with others.
Unfold your own myth.

Rumi

Learn from the mistakes of others.
You can never live long enough
to make them all yourself.

Groucho Marx

_____

_____

_____

_____

_____

_____

_____

_____

_____

_____

_____

_____

_____

_____

—⦿⟨⟩⦿—

I'm going to stand outside.

So, if anyone asks,

I'm outstanding.

Unknown

_____

_____

_____

_____

_____

_____

_____

_____

_____

_____

_____

_____

_____

_____

_____

Change is not a four-letter word ...
but often your reaction to it is!

Jeffrey Gitomer

_____

_____

_____

_____

_____

_____

_____

_____

_____

_____

_____

_____

_____

_____

_____

_____

_____

Dr. Charley Ferrer

Opportunity is missed by most people
because it is dressed in overalls
and looks like work.

Thomas Edison

Opportunity does not knock,
it presents itself when you beat down the door.

Kyle Chandler

_____
_____
_____
_____
_____
_____
_____
_____
_____
_____
_____
_____
_____
_____
_____
_____
_____

A diamond is merely a lump of coal
that did well under pressure.

Unknown

People often say that motivation doesn't
last. Well, neither does bathing
that's why we recommend it daily.

Zig Ziglar

When I hear somebody sigh, "Life is hard,"
I am always tempted to ask,
"Compared to what?"

Sydney Harris

_____

_____

_____

_____

_____

_____

_____

_____

_____

_____

_____

_____

_____

_____

_____

I always wanted to be somebody,
but now I realize
I should have been more specific.

Lilly Tomlin

Well-behaved women
seldom make history.

Laurel Thatcher Ulrich

_____

_____

_____

_____

_____

_____

_____

_____

_____

_____

_____

_____

_____

_____

Take criticism seriously,
but not personally.
If there is truth or merit in the criticism,
try to learn from it.
Otherwise, let it roll right off you.

Hillary Clinton

_____

_____

_____

_____

_____

_____

_____

_____

_____

_____

_____

_____

If you're going to be able to look back on something and laugh about it, you might as well laugh about it now.

Marie Osmond, Singer

_____
_____
_____
_____
_____
_____
_____
_____
_____
_____
_____
_____
_____
_____
_____

I learned to be with myself rather than
avoiding myself with limiting habits;
I started to be aware of my feelings more,
rather than numb them.

Judith Wright

_____

_____

_____

_____

_____

_____

_____

_____

_____

_____

_____

_____

_____

_____

Life is like photography.
You need the negatives to develop.

Unknown

Life is a blank canvas, and you need to
throw all the paint on it you can.

Danny Kaye

_____

_____

_____

_____

_____

_____

_____

_____

_____

_____

_____

_____

_____

_____

_____

_____

_____

If you don't design your own life plan,
chances are you'll fall into someone else's plan.
And guess what they have planned for you?
Not much.

Jim Rohn

———————— ⅱ⟨⟨⟨⟨⟩⟩⟩⟩ⅱ ————————

Life is a shipwreck
but we must not forget
to sing in the lifeboats.

Voltaire, Philosopher

_____

_____

_____

_____

_____

_____

_____

_____

_____

_____

_____

_____

_____

_____

Because true belonging only happens when we present our authentic, imperfect selves to the world, our sense of belonging can never be greater than our level of self-acceptance.

Brené Brown

_____

_____

_____

_____

_____

_____

_____

_____

_____

_____

_____

_____

When we are no longer able to change
a situation, we are challenged
to change ourselves.

Viktor Frankl

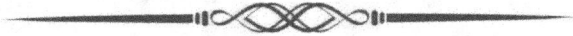

Cherish your visions. Cherish your ideals. Cherish the music that stirs in your heart, the beauty that forms in your mind, the loveliness that drapes your purest thoughts, for out of them will grow all delightful conditions, all heavenly environment, of these, if you but remain true to them your world will at last be built.

As a Man Thinketh
James Allen

_____

_____

_____

_____

_____

_____

_____

_____

_____

_____

Consider the postage stamp:
its usefulness consists in the ability
to stick to one thing 'til it gets there.

Josh Billings

Emotions are temporal—meaning they
need time to exist. Let go and
let the Universe reshape it!

Good things come to those who wait ...
greater things come to those who get off
their ass and do anything to make it happen.

Unknown

_____

_____

_____

_____

_____

_____

_____

_____

_____

_____

_____

_____

_____

_____

_____

_____

———————■○∞◯∞○■———————

I live in the moment.
The moment is the most important thing.
That's my entire philosophy.
Make the best of the good moments.

Rita Moreno

_____

_____

_____

_____

_____

_____

_____

_____

_____

_____

_____

_____

_____

If you can hold onto the bad and angry
thoughts you can do the same to
happy successful thoughts.

Hemal Radia

_____

_____

_____

_____

_____

_____

_____

_____

_____

_____

_____

_____

_____

_____

Don't worry about the world
coming to an end today.
It's already tomorrow in Australia.

Charles Schulz

_____

_____

_____

_____

_____

_____

_____

_____

_____

_____

_____

_____

_____

_____

_____

Here is a test to find whether
your mission on earth is finished:
If you're alive, it isn't.

Richard Bach

_____

_____

_____

_____

_____

_____

_____

_____

_____

_____

_____

_____

_____

_____

_____

_____

Focus, focus, focus!
What am I, a telescope?

Naruto Uzumaki

In essence, if we want to direct our lives,
we must take control of our consistent
actions. It's not what we do once in a while
that shapes our lives,
but what we do consistently.

Tony Robbins

_____

_____

_____

_____

_____

_____

_____

_____

_____

_____

_____

_____

_____

A mountain is composed of tiny
grains of earth. The ocean is made up of
tiny drops of water. Even so, life is but
an endless series of little details, actions,
speeches, and thoughts.
And the consequences whether good or bad
of even the least of them are far-reaching.

Swami Sivananda

_____

_____

_____

_____

_____

_____

_____

_____

_____

_____

_____

Because of your smile,
you make life more beautiful.

Thich Nhat Hanh

———— ıı◇◇◇◇◇ıı ————

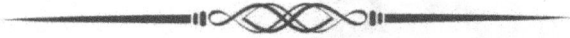

Infuse your life with action. Don't wait for
it to happen. Make it happen. Make your
own future. Make your own hope. Make
your own love. And whatever your beliefs,
honor your creator, not by passively waiting
for grace to come down from upon high, but
by doing what you can to make grace
happen ... yourself, right now,
right down here on earth.

Bradley Whitford

_____

_____

_____

_____

_____

_____

_____

_____

_____

We are all in the gutter,
but some of us are looking at the stars.

Oscar Wilde

_____

_____

_____

_____

_____

_____

_____

_____

_____

_____

_____

_____

_____

_____

_____

_____

_____

No matter how qualified or deserving we
are, we will never reach a better life
until we can imagine it for ourselves
and allow ourselves to have it.

One
Richard Bach

_____

_____

_____

_____

_____

_____

_____

_____

_____

_____

_____

_____

_____

_____

THINK ... it's not illegal yet.

Anonymous

_____

_____

_____

_____

_____

_____

_____

_____

_____

_____

_____

_____

_____

_____

_____

_____

_____

There are far far better things ahead
than any we've left behind.

C.S. Lewis

Evil thrives when good men
[and women] do nothing.

Edmund Burke

_____

_____

_____

_____

_____

_____

_____

_____

_____

_____

_____

_____

_____

_____

_____

_____

———||◇❰✕❱◇||———

Don't make yourself small just so others
will feel comfortable with their mediocrity!

Dr. Charley Ferrer

_____

_____

_____

_____

_____

_____

_____

_____

_____

_____

_____

_____

_____

_____

_____

_____

You get in life what you have
the courage to ask for.

Oprah Winfrey

_____

_____

_____

_____

_____

_____

_____

_____

_____

_____

_____

_____

_____

_____

_____

_____

_____

There are many ways of going forward,
but only one way of standing still.

Franklin D. Roosevelt

_____

_____

_____

_____

_____

_____

_____

_____

_____

_____

_____

_____

_____

_____

_____

_____

Adversity causes some to break
and others to break records.

Nicole Michelle

_____

_____

_____

_____

_____

_____

_____

_____

_____

_____

_____

_____

_____

_____

_____

_____

Every day is a good day
to choose happiness.

Dr. Charley Ferrer

_____

_____

_____

_____

_____

_____

_____

_____

_____

_____

_____

_____

_____

_____

_____

_____

There is inspiration to be found in everything
around us
if we but open our hearts and minds.

Dr. Charley Ferrer

_____

_____

_____

_____

_____

_____

_____

_____

_____

_____

_____

_____

_____

_____

_____

Life is 10% what happens to us
and 90% how we react to it.

Dennis P. Kimbro

_____

_____

_____

_____

_____

_____

_____

_____

_____

_____

_____

_____

_____

_____

There is wonder right in front of us, and we don't spend enough time thinking about it.

Michael Pollan

_____

_____

_____

_____

_____

_____

_____

_____

_____

_____

_____

_____

_____

_____

_____

_____

_____

Doubt is a killer. You just have to know
who you are and what you stand for.

Jennifer Lopez
Actress & Singer

_____
_____
_____
_____
_____
_____
_____
_____
_____
_____
_____
_____
_____

You can be the lead in your own life.

Kerry Washington

_____

_____

_____

_____

_____

_____

_____

_____

_____

_____

_____

_____

_____

_____

_____

_____

Life is much more fun if you live it in the
spirit of play and collaboration,
working with instead of against others.

Wally Amos

_____

_____

_____

_____

_____

_____

_____

_____

_____

_____

_____

_____

_____

_____

_____

The tragedy of life is not that it ends so soon,
but that we wait so long to begin it.

W.M. Lewis

When we speak, we are afraid our words
will not be heard or welcomed.
But when we are silent, we are still afraid.
So, it is better to speak.

Audre Lorde

The quality of a person's life is in direct
proportion to their commitment to
excellence, regardless of their
chosen field of endeavor.

Vince Lombardi

_____

_____

_____

_____

_____

_____

_____

_____

_____

_____

_____

_____

_____

_____

_____

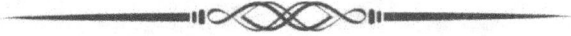

What is required of us is that we love the difficult and learn to deal with it. In the difficult are the friendly forces, the hands that work on us. Right in the difficult we must have our joys, our happiness, our dreams: there against the depth of this background, they stand out, there for the first time we see how beautiful they are.

Rainer Maria Rilke

_____

_____

_____

_____

_____

_____

_____

_____

_____

_____

She was powerful,
not because she wasn't scared
but because she went on so strongly,
despite the fear.

Atticus

_____

_____

_____

_____

_____

_____

_____

_____

_____

_____

_____

_____

_____

_____

—••◦◯◇◯◦••—

Have patience with all things.
But most importantly,
have patience with yourself.

Saint Frances de Sales

_____

_____

_____

_____

_____

_____

_____

_____

_____

_____

_____

_____

_____

Owning our story can be hard
but not nearly as difficult
as spending our lives running from it.

Brené Brown

_____
_____
_____
_____
_____
_____
_____
_____
_____
_____
_____
_____
_____
_____
_____

The most precious thing
that we all have with us is time.

Steve Jobs

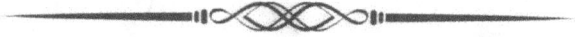

In the end it's not which path you've
taken, it's why you choose it.

Dr. Charley Ferrer

_____

_____

_____

_____

_____

_____

_____

_____

_____

_____

_____

_____

_____

_____

_____

_____

_____

Sometimes the hardest thing isn't letting go, it's learning to start over.

Nicole Savon

Make today so awesome
that yesterday gets jealous!

Anonymous

I have less fear of dying,
than I do of not living.

Unknown

You have trust in what you think.
If you splinter yourself and try to please
everyone, you can't.

Annie Leibovitz

_____

_____

_____

_____

_____

_____

_____

_____

_____

_____

_____

_____

_____

_____

_____

If someone tells you you can't do something, don't get discouraged just show them five ways to do it.

Unknown

_____

_____

_____

_____

_____

_____

_____

_____

_____

_____

_____

_____

If your mind is cluttered,
how will you hear
what your heart has to say?

Unknown

_____

_____

_____

_____

_____

_____

_____

_____

_____

_____

_____

_____

_____

_____

_____

What's right isn't always popular.
What's popular isn't always right.

H. Jackson Brown, Jr.

_____

_____

_____

_____

_____

_____

_____

_____

_____

_____

_____

_____

_____

_____

_____

When you really discover life is limitless,
what will you do with it?

Dr. Charley Ferrer

_____

_____

_____

_____

_____

_____

_____

_____

_____

_____

_____

_____

_____

_____

_____

_____

_____

_____

_____

━━━━━━━━◊◊◊◊━━━━━━━━

Sometimes you're a "sugar cookie"
because life is not fair.

Make Your Bed
Colonel William H. McRaven

_____

_____

_____

_____

_____

_____

_____

_____

_____

_____

_____

_____

_____

_____

_____

_____

Do you want to meet the love of your life?
Look in the mirror.

Byron Katie

_____

_____

_____

_____

_____

_____

_____

_____

_____

_____

_____

_____

_____

_____

_____

Magic is everywhere. Find yours.

Give a girl the right pair of shoes
and she'll conquer the world.

Marilyn Monroe

Stop Surviving and Start THRIVING!

Breast Cancer
9 Essentials to Navigate Cancer
Dr. Charley Ferrer

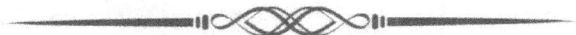

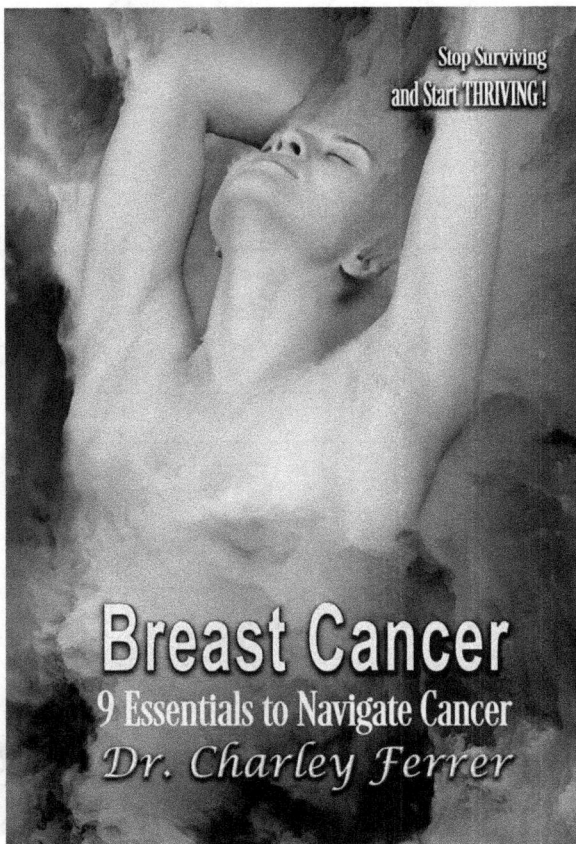

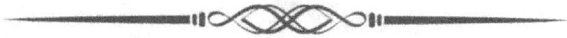

It has been said that everyone dies

but not everyone lives.

How will you choose to live the time
you have left?

Will you do so in anger and sadness,
or in adventurous wonder
of all you can experience before you leave this
plain of existence?

Dr. Charley Ferrer

Stop sleeping on your dreams
and act on them!

_____

_____

_____

_____

_____

_____

_____

_____

_____

_____

_____

_____

_____

_____

_____

_____

De ilusión también se vive.

You can also live on illusions—dreams.

Spanish Proverb
Interpreted many different ways

_____

_____

_____

_____

_____

_____

_____

_____

_____

_____

_____

_____

_____

_____

_____

When things are bad,
it's the best time to reinvent yourself.

George Lopez

What if this universe is merely a dream?

Dr. Charley Ferrer

Life is not a fairy tale. If you lose your
shoe at midnight, you're drunk.

Unknown

_____
_____
_____
_____
_____
_____
_____
_____
_____
_____
_____
_____
_____
_____
_____

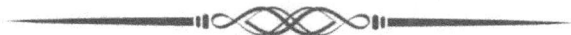

Make the most of yourself by fanning
the tiny, inner sparks of possibility
into flames of achievement.

Golda Meir

_____

_____

_____

_____

_____

_____

_____

_____

_____

_____

_____

_____

_____

_____

_____

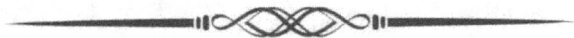

Beauty is everywhere. Aim Happy.

Unknown

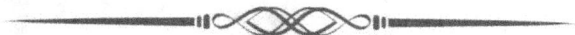

You have a glass there's something in it.

If you like what it is, add more.

If you don't, pour it out and start again.

F**k it if the glass is empty or full.

That doesn't matter.

What really matters is,

are you gonna do something about it,

with it, or not!

Tim S. Grover

_____

_____

_____

_____

_____

_____

_____

_____

_____

_____

Do you want to be the hero
or the hero's girlfriend?

Plum's question in Dietland
Sarai Walker

_____
_____
_____
_____
_____
_____
_____
_____
_____
_____
_____
_____
_____
_____
_____
_____

You're blazing a trail not following one.

Gary John Bishop

_____

_____

_____

_____

_____

_____

_____

_____

_____

_____

_____

_____

_____

_____

_____

_____

_____

‖⟨⟩‖

Accept. Modify. Improve.

_____

_____

_____

_____

_____

_____

_____

_____

_____

_____

_____

_____

_____

_____

_____

_____

_____

_____

F**k how you feel. Act!

_____
_____
_____
_____
_____
_____
_____
_____
_____
_____
_____
_____
_____
_____
_____
_____
_____
_____
_____

Don't let cancer dictate your reality.

Dr. Charley Ferrer

_____

_____

_____

_____

_____

_____

_____

_____

_____

_____

_____

_____

_____

_____

_____

_____

_____

_____

_____

Expect nothing and accept everything.

Gary John Bishop

_____

_____

_____

_____

_____

_____

_____

_____

_____

_____

_____

_____

_____

_____

_____

_____

Don't all roads lead to sex?

Dr. Charley Ferrer

_____

_____

_____

_____

_____

_____

_____

_____

_____

_____

_____

_____

_____

_____

_____

I'd rather regret the things I've done than
regret the things I haven't done.

Lucille Ball

_____

_____

_____

_____

_____

_____

_____

_____

_____

_____

_____

_____

_____

_____

_____

_____

_____

Never feel bad to demand your worth for
your work and the services you provide.

Dr. Isaura Gonzalez

_____

_____

_____

_____

_____

_____

_____

_____

_____

_____

_____

_____

_____

_____

_____

_____

She believed that she could ... so she did!

"Dictate the Tempo"

Unknown

_____
_____
_____
_____
_____
_____
_____
_____
_____
_____
_____
_____
_____
_____
_____

Carry out a random act of kindness,
with no expectation of reward,
safe in the knowledge that one day
someone might do the same for you.

Diana
Princess of Wales

Men make the moral code and they expect
women to accept it. They have decided that
it is entirely right and proper for men to
fight for their liberties and their rights,
but that it is not right or proper
for women to fight for theirs.

Emmeline Pankhurst
1858 – 1928

_____

_____

_____

_____

_____

_____

_____

_____

_____

_____

_____

_____

The more you have,
the more you have to give.

Hugh Jackson, Actor

_____
_____
_____
_____
_____
_____
_____
_____
_____
_____
_____
_____
_____
_____
_____
_____
_____

No one ever made a difference
being like everybody else.

P.T. Barnum

_____

_____

_____

_____

_____

_____

_____

_____

_____

_____

_____

_____

_____

_____

_____

_____

The new you is the old you
before the world got you down.

The Sell
Fredrik Eklund

_____

_____

_____

_____

_____

_____

_____

_____

_____

_____

_____

_____

_____

_____

_____

Don't go around saying the world owes you
a living. The world owes you nothing.
It was here first.

Mark Twain

_____
_____
_____
_____
_____
_____
_____
_____
_____
_____
_____
_____
_____
_____
_____
_____
_____

[Life] isn't a dress rehearsal.

Waylon Jennings

Don't talk yourself out of
what God wants for you.

Joel Osteen

_____
_____
_____
_____
_____
_____
_____
_____
_____
_____
_____
_____
_____
_____
_____
_____
_____
_____

To what extremes would you go to bring
about your heart's fondest wishes,
to manifest your greatest desires, and to live
your boldest dreams? OMG - Did you just
say visualize daily and take baby steps?!

Notes from The Universe
Mike Dooley

Rehearse your victories.

Joel Osteen

_____

_____

_____

_____

_____

_____

_____

_____

_____

_____

_____

_____

_____

_____

_____

_____

_____

_____

We all die, so what excuse are you using
not to live to your full potential ...
your full adventure ... your full life?

Dr. Charley Ferrer

_____

_____

_____

_____

_____

_____

_____

_____

_____

_____

_____

_____

_____

_____

This isn't who you are,
it's just the job you're doing on
the road to who you want to be.

_____

_____

_____

_____

_____

_____

_____

_____

_____

_____

_____

_____

_____

_____

_____

_____

_____

Make progress not perfection.

Movie — The Equalizer

_____

_____

_____

_____

_____

_____

_____

_____

_____

_____

_____

_____

_____

_____

_____

_____

_____

Life is uncertain...eat dessert first.

Ernestine Ulmer

Wouldn't it be great to say to yourself,
"I'm going to be AWESOME today because I was
F**KING FABULOUS yesterday!"

Dr. Charley Ferrer

_____

_____

_____

_____

_____

_____

_____

_____

_____

_____

_____

_____

_____

_____

Don't underestimate your influence!

_____

_____

_____

_____

_____

_____

_____

_____

_____

_____

_____

_____

_____

_____

_____

_____

_____

_____

Are you the woman (man)
you want to see in the mirror?

Dr. Charley Ferrer

_____

_____

_____

_____

_____

_____

_____

_____

_____

_____

_____

_____

_____

_____

_____

_____

_____

You can never see further
than the choices you're willing to make.

Unknown

_____

_____

_____

_____

_____

_____

_____

_____

_____

_____

_____

_____

_____

_____

_____

_____

I was exhilarated by the new realization
that I could change the character of my life
by changing my beliefs.

Bruce Lipton

_____

_____

_____

_____

_____

_____

_____

_____

_____

_____

_____

_____

_____

_____

———————— ⅱ◇◇◇ⅱ ————————

What I know now is that when it feels like
shit, that means that I am being fertilized
to help me grow.

Co-Dependence:
The Dance of the Wounded Soul
Robert Burney

_____

_____

_____

_____

_____

_____

_____

_____

_____

_____

_____

_____

_____

_____

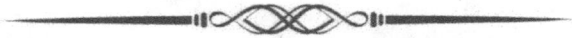

I wanted a perfect ending.
Now I've learned, the hard way,
that some poems don't rhyme, and some
stories don't have a clear beginning, middle,
and end. Life is about not knowing,
having to change, taking the moment and
making the best of it, without knowing
what's going to happen next.
Delicious Ambiguity.

Gilda Radner

Circumstances don't make the man,
They reveal him to himself.

Epictetus
Circa 55 – 135 AD

_____

_____

_____

_____

_____

_____

_____

_____

_____

_____

_____

_____

_____

_____

_____

_____

———||◦⟨✕⟩◦||———

It's no use going back to yesterday because
I was a different person then.

Alice in Wonderland
Lewis Carroll

_____

_____

_____

_____

_____

_____

_____

_____

_____

_____

_____

_____

_____

_____

_____

_____

⸺‖◦◦◇◇◦◦‖⸺

Live and love beyond what you think is
possible. Demand it all ... want it all.
Reach for the universe!
You'll be amazed at what happens next.

Thought inspired by Gary John Bishop
Dr. Charley Ferrer

_____

_____

_____

_____

_____

_____

_____

_____

_____

_____

_____

_____

_____

_____

_____

—||◦◦⟨⟨✕⟩⟩◦◦||—

If you think you can or you think you can't,
you're right.

Henry Ford

_____
_____
_____
_____
_____
_____
_____
_____
_____
_____
_____
_____
_____
_____
_____

You don't need to destroy your life
—nor accept hardship—
just to make others happy.

Dr. Charley Ferrer

_____

_____

_____

_____

_____

_____

_____

_____

_____

_____

_____

_____

_____

_____

_____

As long as you feed the beast, it will live.

Jen Sincero

Before getting out of bed,
set your mind for victory.
Set your mind for success.
Otherwise, you allow negativity to set in.

Joel Osteen

_____

_____

_____

_____

_____

_____

_____

_____

_____

_____

_____

_____

_____

_____

—————————⊪◯⬦⬦◯⊪—————————

We realize the importance of our voices
only when we are silenced.

Malala Yousafzai

_____

_____

_____

_____

_____

_____

_____

_____

_____

_____

_____

_____

_____

_____

Victory loves preparation.

The Movie: Mechanic

Create the change you want to see in life.

Mahatma Gandhi

_____

_____

_____

_____

_____

_____

_____

_____

_____

_____

_____

_____

_____

_____

_____

_____

_____

I pray you, do not fall in love with me
for I am falser than vows made in wine.

As You Like It
Shakespeare

_____

_____

_____

_____

_____

_____

_____

_____

_____

_____

_____

_____

_____

_____

_____

_____

_____

Expect more from yourself than anyone
else can ever expect from you.

Michael Jordan

_____

_____

_____

_____

_____

_____

_____

_____

_____

_____

_____

_____

_____

_____

_____

Do not go where the path may lead
—go instead where there is no path—
and leave a trail.

Ralph Waldo Emerson

_____

_____

_____

_____

_____

_____

_____

_____

_____

_____

_____

_____

_____

_____

———||∞⟨⟩∞||———

Sometimes you have to serve in order to lead.

Odysseys

_____
_____
_____
_____
_____
_____
_____
_____
_____
_____
_____
_____
_____
_____
_____
_____
_____
_____

Never allow someone to be your priority
while allowing yourself to be their option.

Ariane Rubio

_____

_____

_____

_____

_____

_____

_____

_____

_____

_____

_____

_____

_____

_____

_____

_____

Just as the great oceans have but one taste,
the taste of salt, so too there is but one taste
fundamental to all true teachings of the
ways, and this is the taste of freedom.

Buddha

_____
_____
_____
_____
_____
_____
_____
_____
_____
_____
_____
_____
_____

What you feel only matters to you.
What you do is what matters
to the people you love.

Dr. Charley Ferrer

_____

_____

_____

_____

_____

_____

_____

_____

_____

_____

_____

_____

_____

_____

_____

Ultimately, a hero is a man who would
argue with the gods and awaken the devils
to contest his vision.

Norman Mailer

_____

_____

_____

_____

_____

_____

_____

_____

_____

_____

_____

_____

_____

_____

_____

_____

_____

_____

Seduce my mind and you can have my body.
Find my soul and I'm yours forever.

Anonymous

Discipline is the bridge
between learning and accomplishment.

Jim Rohn

Sometimes when you stare long into the Abyss
... the abyss stares into you.

Friedrich Nietzsche

_____

_____

_____

_____

_____

_____

_____

_____

_____

_____

_____

_____

_____

_____

_____

_____

_____

_____

Nearly all men can stand adversity,
but if you want to test a man's character,
give him power.

Abraham Lincoln

My bed is a magical place
where I suddenly remember
everything I forgot to do.

Cool Funny Quotes

_____

_____

_____

_____

_____

_____

_____

_____

_____

_____

_____

_____

_____

_____

_____

_____

———— ₪∽⟨⟨✕⟩⟩∾₪ ————

Pain is inevitable. Suffering is optional!

M. Kathleen Casey

_____

_____

_____

_____

_____

_____

_____

_____

_____

_____

_____

_____

_____

_____

_____

_____

Scars remind us where we've been,
they don't have to dictate
where you're going.

David Rossi

_____

_____

_____

_____

_____

_____

_____

_____

_____

_____

_____

_____

_____

_____

_____

_____

A coward dies a thousand deaths,
the brave men only once.

William Shakespeare

Feet?
Why do I need them
when I have wings to fly!

Frida Kahlo

_____

_____

_____

_____

_____

_____

_____

_____

_____

_____

_____

_____

_____

_____

_____

_____

Focus on where you want to go
not what you fear.

Anthony Robbins

Love is a gift you give to yourself;
others merely benefit from it.

Dr. Charley Ferrer

_____

_____

_____

_____

_____

_____

_____

_____

_____

_____

_____

_____

_____

_____

_____

_____

_____

Only those that can see the invisible
can do the impossible.

Albert Einstein

The butterfly counts not months
but moments, and has time enough.

Rabindranath Tagore

Knowing yourself
is the beginning of all wisdom.

_____

_____

_____

_____

_____

_____

_____

_____

_____

_____

_____

_____

_____

_____

_____

_____

_____

_____

There are always flowers
for those who see them.

Henri Matisse

_____

_____

_____

_____

_____

_____

_____

_____

_____

_____

_____

_____

_____

_____

_____

_____

_____

———||∞⟨⟩∞||———

Hills are always more beautiful
than stone buildings.

Walking Buffalo

_____
_____
_____
_____
_____
_____
_____
_____
_____
_____
_____
_____
_____
_____
_____
_____

The wildness is the
preservation of the world.

Henry David Thoreau

_____

_____

_____

_____

_____

_____

_____

_____

_____

_____

_____

_____

_____

_____

_____

_____

_____

Ask yourself, "Is this the reality
I want to live?" If the answer is no,
start to change it.

Dr. Charley Ferrer

_____

_____

_____

_____

_____

_____

_____

_____

_____

_____

_____

_____

_____

_____

There is no life as complete
as the life that is lived by choice.

Shad Helmstetter

_____

_____

_____

_____

_____

_____

_____

_____

_____

_____

_____

_____

_____

_____

_____

_____

_____

_____

Nothing ever becomes real
'til it is experienced.

John Keats

I've got a great ambition to die of
exhaustion rather than boredom.

Thomas Carlyle

_____
_____
_____
_____
_____
_____
_____
_____
_____
_____
_____
_____
_____
_____
_____
_____
_____

I am not what happened to me,
I am what I choose to become.

C.G. Jung

_____

_____

_____

_____

_____

_____

_____

_____

_____

_____

_____

_____

_____

_____

_____

_____

Do you know the difference between
education and experience?
Education is when you read the fine print;
experience is what you get when you don't.

Pete Seeger

_____

_____

_____

_____

_____

_____

_____

_____

_____

_____

_____

_____

_____

———————=ll◦∞◯∞◦ll=———————

After you've done a thing the same way for
two years, look it over carefully. After five
years, look at it with suspicion. And after ten
years, throw it away and start all over.

Alfred Edward Perlman

When the winds of change blow,
some people build walls
and others build windmills.

Chinese Proverb

_____
_____
_____
_____
_____
_____
_____
_____
_____
_____
_____
_____
_____
_____
_____
_____
_____

I didn't get there by wishing for it
or hoping for it, but by working for it.

Estée Lauder

I am not afraid of storms
for I am learning how to sail my ship.

Louisa May Alcott

_____

_____

_____

_____

_____

_____

_____

_____

_____

_____

_____

_____

_____

_____

_____

_____

You're a human being,
you live once and life is wonderful;
so eat the damn red velvet cupcake.

Emma Stone

One is not born a woman;
one becomes one.

Simone De Deauvoir

_____

_____

_____

_____

_____

_____

_____

_____

_____

_____

_____

_____

_____

_____

_____

_____

_____

_____

_____

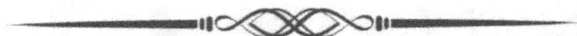

To attract better you have to
become better yourself.

You can't do the same things
and expect change.

You can't blame anyone
or anything.

It's time to take responsibility
for your reality.

Start transforming your mindset.

Start upgrading your habits.

Start being more positive.

Idil Ahmed

I didn't know what I wanted to do but I always knew the woman I wanted to be.

Diane von Furstenberg

If I stop to kick every barking dog
I am not going to get where I'm going.

Jackie Joyner-Kersee

_____

_____

_____

_____

_____

_____

_____

_____

_____

_____

_____

_____

_____

_____

_____

_____

You are the one that possesses the keys to
your being. You carry the passport to your
own happiness.

Diane von Furstenberg

I was smart enough to go through
any door that opened.

Joan Rivers

_____

_____

_____

_____

_____

_____

_____

_____

_____

_____

_____

_____

_____

_____

_____

Power's not given to you.
You have to take it.

Beyoncé Knowles Carter

_____

_____

_____

_____

_____

_____

_____

_____

_____

_____

_____

_____

_____

_____

_____

I tried to drown my sorrows,
but the bastards learned how to swim,
and now I am overwhelmed
by this decent and good feeling.

Frida Kahlo

If you plan it ... life happens.

Dr. Charley Ferrer

Books by Dr. Charley Ferrer

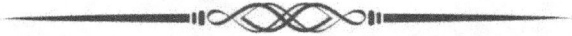

Breast Cancer: From Diagnosis to Surgery
Breast Cancer 9 Essentials to Navigate
Cancer
The W.I.S.E. Journal for the Sensual Woman
Sex AFTER Cancer (coming soon)

Breast Cancer Diaries Series

Inspirational Quotes, Thoughts and
Comments
Choose
Breast Cancer Diaries
Breast Cancer Diaries -- The Play
Things to Do While You Wait

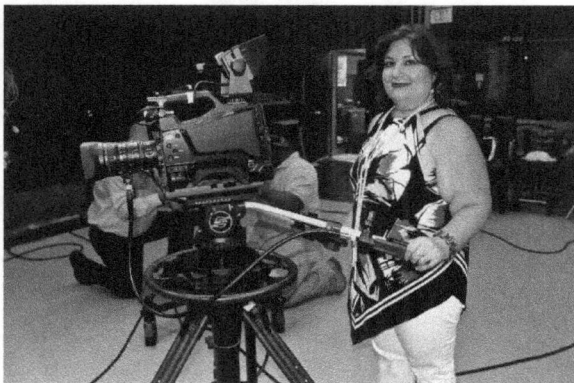

Dr. Charley Ferrer is a world-renowned Clinical Sexologist and award-winning author. She has lectured throughout the U.S., Latin America and China on sexual health and self-empowerment for the past twenty years.

After being diagnosed with breast cancer, she turned her fears and frustrations at the lack of medical information provided to cancer patients into a popular television series. She established the Cancer Tamer Foundation, a non-profit 501(c)(3) organizations that provides women with

—————ᴵᴵᦆ⬤⬤ᦆᴵᴵ—————

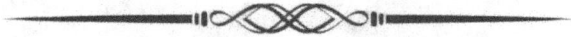

cancer with education, supportive services, and
life-enriching activities. Cancer Tamer is a new
voice in the "war" against cancer.

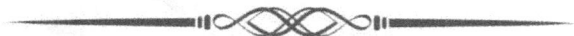

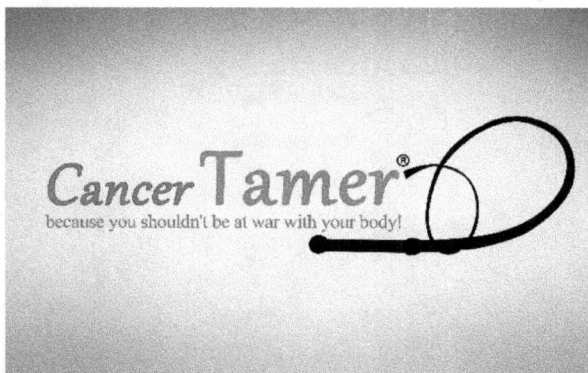

www.CancerTamer.org